THE BOWEL NOSODES

THE BOWEL NOSODES

BY

JOHN PATERSON

M. B., Ch. B., D. P. H. (Camb.), F. F. Hom. Presented by Médi-T.

KALPAZ

ISBN: 978-93-5128-550-2

First Published in 1949
Indian Reprint in 2017

Published by

Kalpaz Publications
C-30, Satyawati Nagar,
Delhi – 110052
E-mail: kalpaz@hotmail.com
Website: kalpazpublications.com
Ph.: +91-9212142040

Cataloging in Publication Data—DK
Courtesy: D.K. Agencies (P) Ltd. <docinfo@dkagencies.com>

Paterson, John, 1890-1954, **author.**
The bowel nosodes / by John Paterson.
pages cm
"First published in 1949"—Title page verso.
ISBN 9789351285502

1. Homeopathy—Materia medica and therapeutics. 2. Bacterial vaccines. I. Title.

RX601.P38 2017 DDC 615.532 23

INTRODUCTION

The name of one of your illustrious countrymen, Louis Pasteur, will forever be remembered as the founder of the science of bacteriology. It was he who first isolated and identified a specific germ and related it to a definite clinical entity (disease). Following upon his discoveries, medical science concentrated on the laboratory technique for the isolation and identification of a specific germ for each known disease, and the Koch postulates were accepted as the standard for declaring any germ capable of pathogenesis -of having power to cause disease. The motto of the medical profession is still *Tolle Causam,* find the cause, and to-day there are many who consider that germs are the only cause of disease and are working to discover the specific germ or virus for well known clinical entities.

It must now be accepted as scientific fact that specific germs, in many cases of disease can be isolated and identified, but is it a true conclusion that the specific germ is always the cause of the disease ? The subject is too great to be dealt with in all its aspects in this short session, but a little time must be given to considering the general question, namely the role of the Bacterium in Nature because one's opinion on this must determine the value one places on the use of bacterial products -vaccines or nosodes- in the treatment of disease. As the subject of this paper deals with the intestinal flora, I propose to limit my remarks to consideration of the role played by the *B. Coli* and coliform organisms found in the intestinal tract.

The role of the intestinal bacteria. B. Coli can be isolated from the intestine of all warm blooded animals and have been found on grasses outside the body, where there seemed to be no possibility of faecal contamination. Most workers consider the B.

* Read to the Rhodacienne Homœopathic Society at the meeting of the International Homœopathic League Council, August, 1949. *Coli* to be a *harmless* saprophyte and to be non-pathogenic in the healthy bowel. Its function is to break up into the more simple substances the complex molecules of the organic combinations, which form the bodies of plants and animals, or of the complex substances which result from the digestive processes in the intestinal canal and are excreted. It is important to note this function in the further study of the intestinal flora and its relationship to disease.

In nature, where there is balance, there is no *disease* and the germ, in this case the *B. Coli* in the intestinal tract, performs a useful function. Where the intestinal mucosa is healthy the *B. Coli* is non-pathogenic. Any change in the host which affects the intestinal mucosa will upset the balance and will be followed by a change in the habit and the bio-chemistry of the *B. Coli,* which may then be said to become pathogenic, but it should be noted that the primary change, the disease originated in the host, which compelled the bacillus to modify its habit in order to survive. I would ask you to keep this sequence of events in mind as a great deal of what I have to say about the intestinal nosodes is based upon this conception which I have confirmed by clinical and laboratory observations over the last twenty years.

In 1936 I presented a paper to the British Homœopathic Society, which was published in their *Journal* of April 1936, under the title of "The potentized Drug and Its Action on the Bowel Flora" and it dealt with the clinical and bacteriological observations on 12,000 cases. A brief summary of the findings is as follows:

(a) Non-lactose fermenting bacilli were isolated in 25 per cent. of the stool specimens examined.

(b) The appearance of non-lactose fermenting bacilli often *followed* and seemed to bear relationship to the previously administered homœopathic remedy -the choice of the remedy being made according to "the law of similars" and prepared by "potentization".

In the laboratory one observed an unexpected phenomenon, that from a patient who had previously yielded only *B. Coli* there suddenly appeared a large percentage of non-lactose fermenting bacilli of a type which. One associated with the pathogenic group of typhoid and paratyphoid.

If one accepts the view, generally held, that the *B. Coli* of the intestinal tract is a harmless saprophyte and is non-pathogenic it must be concluded that, so far as the intestinal tract was concerned there was no evidence of disease in these patients during the first series of examinations. Now the patient's stool yielded a large percentage of presumably pathogenic organisms, and according to the accepted Pasteur and Koch theory, the patient was suffering from disease. Clinical investigations, however, revealed that the patient did not feel ill, but had experienced a sense of well being which he had attributed to the last medicine he had received. Since the non-lactose fermenting bacilli had appeared after a definite latent period of 10 to '4 days, following the administration of the remedy, it would seem that the homsopathic *potentized remedy* had changed the bowel flora, and had caused the disease. The pathogenic germ in this case was the *result* of vital action set up in the patient by the potentized remedy. The germ was *not* the cause of the disease.

Is the "specific germ" the actual cause of disease, or is it the result of the action of the vital force (Dynamis) which characterises all living cells, in their resistance to *disease ?* That is a question which I must ask you to consider and answer for yourselves in the light of the observations I have placed before you today. Meantime, it will be sufficient for the purpose of continuing the subject of this paper, if we agree that each germ is associated with its own peculiar symptom picture (disease) and that certain conclusions may be made from these clinical and laboratory observations and translated into the practice of medicine.

(a) The specific organism is related to the disease.

(b) The specific organism is *related to the homś opathic remedy.*

(c) The homœopathic remedy is related to the disease.

From my observations I have been able to compile a list of bowel organisms with their related homœopathic remedies and to associate a clinical picture i. e. to offer a "proving" for each type of bowel organism. In this case the word "proving" is not used in the strict Hahnemannian sense-experiment on the healthy human -but on clinical observation of the sick person.

It is not possible to give a detailed account of each type in one session, so I propose to give you a brief summary for each, indicating a keynote, the main action. From this, and your knowledge of the associated homœopathic remedies, you should be able to formulate a more complete picture of the symptom complex of these bowel organisms, and later I shall indicate how this knowledge can be put into practice.

MORGAN (Bach)

B. MORGAN is the type of non lactose organism most frequently found in the stool and it has the greatest number of associated remedies compared to other types on the list.

The keynote for the *Morgan* group is contained in the word "*Congestion*" and if this is used in the study of the various parts of the body affected it will afford a good symptom picture of the pathogenesis of the *B. Morgan.*

Head. Congestive headaches, with flushed face; worse from hot atmosphere; thundery weather; excitement; travelling in bus or train. Vertigo from high blood pressure.

Mentals. Introspective, anxious and apprehensive about state of health; irritability; avoids company but often shows mental anxiety if left alone. Mental depression, often with suicidal tendency.

Digestive System. Congestion of gastric mucosa and liver; heart-burn pyrosis, dirty tongue, bitter taste in mouth in the morning with accumulation of mucus causing gagging as soon as rises from bed. Congestion of liver; "bilious attacks" with severe headache which is finally relieved by vomiting large quantities of bile stained mucus. (A history of "bilious attacks', especially occurring at the menopause in women should lead one to consider the use of the nosode, *Morgan* (Bach).) Cholecystitis, gallstone; constipation, hæmorrhoids, pruritus ani.

Respiratory System. Congestion of nasal and bronchial membrane, especially in children, broncho- and lobar pneumonia. (A history of repeated attacks of "congestion of the lungs" or broncho-pneumonia, in children, is indicative for the use of the nosode *Morgan* (Bach) or one of the sub-types *Morgan-pure* (Paterson) or *Morgan-Gaertner* (Paterson).)

It is worth noticing, in view of the frequent use of the Sulpha drugs in the treatment of pneumonia, that *Sulphur* is outstanding among the remedies associated with *Bacillus Morgan* of the intestinal tract.

Genito-urinary System. The congestive headache associated with the menstrual onset has already been mentioned, and this is often accompanied by ovarian pain (congestive dysmenorrhœa) or by the congestive flushings of the menopause period.

Circulation. Congestion and sluggish action is seen by the tendency to hemorrhoids and varicose veins and the condition known as "Erythro cyanosis puellorum", a blueness of the lower extremities, often in female adolescents and marked by chilblains of feet and toes.

Fibrous Tissues. Chronic congestion around the joints causes arthritic conditions, usually affecting the phalangeal or knee joint regions.

Skin. It is here that the outstanding action of the *Bacillus Morgan* group of organisms is to be found. *Morgan* (Bach) is the nosode indicated where there is congestion of the skin with itching eruption, worse from heat. The type of eruption which characterises this can be ascertained from a study of the "provings" of well known skin remedies found among the list of remedies associated with the *Bacillus Morgan,* e. g. *Sulphur, Graphites, Petroleum* and *Psorinum.* There are few eczemas of the infant at the teething stage or later life, which do not require a dose of this nosode *Morgan* (Bach). It was found possible to isolate two sub-types of *Bacillus Morgan* and to observe the clinical indications for the use of the respective nosodes.

1. *MORGAN-PURE* (Paterson) is indicated where there is a marked symptom of skin eruption or disturbance of the liver; bilious headache, or actual presence of gallstones.
2. *MORGAN-GAERTNER* (Paterson) is also indicated in skin and liver conditions, but it is likely to be more useful where there is evidence of acute inflammatory attack, such as that found in Cholecystitis.

The sub-type *Morgan-Gaertner* (Paterson) has often been found in the stool of patients suffering from renal colic and where X-ray has demonstrated the presence of renal calculus. The nosode *Morgan-Gaertner* (Paterson) should therefore be considered as a possible remedy in cases of renal colic. It is also likely to be of value in treatment in any case which has 4-8 p. m. modality which is also a characteristic of the group prototype *remedy-Lycopodium.* For its prototype, *Morgan-Pure* (Paterson) has *Sulphur* and within the main group represented by *Morgan* (Bach) you will find the well known trio of remedies mentioned by Kent as working in a cycle of *Sulphur, Calcarea Carbonica* and *Lycopodium.*

ROTEUS (Bach)

It is difficult to offer you a single word with which to explain the pathogenesis of the *B. Proteus,* but it will be useful at the outset to suggest to you that the nosode *Proteus* (Bach) will seldom have any therapeutic action unless there are outstanding symptoms in the case relative to the central or peripheral nervous systems and symptoms which appear with degree of suddenness.

Mentals. Mental symptoms are prominent in the clinical proving and "Brain Storm" might be taken as the keynote to indicate this sudden and violent upset of the nervous system.

Outburst of violent temper, specially if opposed in any way; will throw any missile which is at hand; kick or strike; the child objecting to parental control will lie on the floor and kick and scream.

Emotional hysteria, suggestive of the remedy *Ignatia* is also found in the proving of this *B. Proteus* preparation and convulsive and epileptiform seizures and meningismus in children during febrile attacks often responds to the action of the nosode *Proteus* (Bach). Further indication for the use of this nosode is disturbance of the peripheral nervous system, evidenced by *spasm* of the peripheral circulation, e. g. "dead fingers intermittent claudication in the circulation of the lower limbs; anginal attacks due to spasm of the coronary capillaries. There are two well known diseases associated with capillary spasm where the nosode *Proteus* (Bach) has been found useful in treatment-Raynaud's Disease, where there is spasm of the capillary circulation of the extremities, and Meniere's Disease where spasm of the brain circulation results in vertigo attacks.

Digestive System. It is important to note that any of the symptoms manifest in the digestive system are secondary to the action of the central nervous system. It is now being realised that prolonged nerve strain is a factor in the production of duodenal ulcer, and in the' *Proteus* proving, this is also to be found. The type of case is that where there are no prodromal symptoms in the digestive system and the first sign is that of a hæmatemesis or melæna. These ulcers have a tendency to perforate, probably due to the enervation and interference with capillary circulation in that area.

As part of the scientific discussion at this meeting, a study is to be made of the remedy *Natrum muriaticum* and you will note that this is given in my list as the outstanding member of the list of remedies I associate with the *Proteus* nosode, and I may have the opportunity of further discussing with you the significance of the disturbed chloride metabolism associated with this intestinal organism.

Neuromuscular System. As one might expect from the foregoing indications, cramp of muscles is a characteristic symptom and *Cuprum metallicum* is also found among the list of remedies.

Skin. Angio-neurotic œdema, which one associates with the remedy *Apis mellifica* is found in the proving of the *B. Proteus* preparation and also a tendency for the production of herpetic eruption at the mucocutaneous margins.

There is marked sensitivity to exposure to ultra-violet light.

Before leaving this "proving" of *Proteus* (Bach), it may be of interest to you to know that in Great Britain since the war years, there has been a marked increase in the frequency with which one has been able to isolate *B. Proteus,* and this I associate with long continued "nerve strain"-a factor of considerable importance of the pathogenesis of this type of bowel organism.

BACILLUS No. "7" (Paterson)

This is so named because it was the $_7$th non-lactose fermenting type of bacillus to be observed in the laboratory, and as it did not conform to any of the previously known groups, it was given the numeral "7".

As a keynote for the use of this nosode I suggest *"Mental and Physical Fatigue"*. The "proving" of *Bacillus No.* "7" is not unlike that of *Proteus* (Bach) as it has similar relationship; *Proteus* (Bach) is related to *Chlorine* whereas *Bacillus No.* "7" seems to have a closer relationship to the two halogens, *Bromine* and *iodine,* often in combination with *Potassium.*

Mentals. The outstanding symptom is mental fatigue, a feeling of unfitness for any mental effort, which produces a sense of extreme physical exhaustion.

Digestive System. All the symptoms can be related to general lack of nerve and muscle tone; a sense of fullness after food; flatulence and distension of the stomach; enteroptosis.

Genito-urinary System. Feeble urinary flow; loss of sexual function, premature senility.

Respiratory System. Asthma; bronchial catarrh; tough sticky mucus, difficult to raise.

(Compare the symptom picture of *Kali carb.,* which is one of the associated remedies.)

Circulation. Slow pulse rate, often with lowered blood pressure; myocardial weakness.

(Potassium has a specific action on cardiac muscle.)

Neuro-muscular System. Relaxed fibrous tissue, with tendency to the formation of "rheumatic nodules"; backache, cannot stand long without feeling of faintness; tendency to syncope after sudden exertion.

Skin. Nothing outstanding; sensitive to cold, to draughts and cold damp air.

GAERTNER (Bach)

The keynote for this nosode is *"malnutrition"* and as this would imply, it is the nosode applicable to the treatment of many diseases of childhood, but it is also found to be of value in the other extreme of life associated with malignancy. Marked emaciation may be taken as an indication for the use of the *Gaertner* nosode.

Mentals. Mostly observed in the child; hypersensitive to all impressions, psychical or physical; overactive brain with under-nourished body.

Digestion. It is in the digestive tract that the *B. Gaertner* has its greatest action, and this often manifests itself about the age of 6 months at the time when the infant is put on to artificial feeding.

The inability to digest *fat -cś liac disease; ketosis; "intestinal infantilism" - are all* disease complexes found under the "proving" of the *B. Gaertner* preparations; also *chronic gastro-enteritis; tabes mesenterica;* threadworms. The clearing of threadworms is difficult and usually requires prolonged treatment.

If you combine the clinical picture of three well known remedies with which you are familiar, *Phosphorus, Silicea, Merc. viv.,* you will have before you a very good clinical picture of the "proving" of *Gaertner* (Bach).

DYS. CO. (Bach)

This is the nosode prepared from *B. Dysenterir̹* and the keynote for its use is nervous *tension* of a peculiar type and best described as *"anticipatory",* since it is that sense of nerve tension which a student might feel immediately before facing his examiners, or a business man before attending an important engagement.

Mentals. Nervous tension, mental uneasiness in anticipation of some event; hypersensitive to criticism; shyness and uneasiness among strangers; mental uneasiness shows itself by physical restlessness, cannot keep still, fidgets, choreic movements of facial muscles, or limbs. Headache, frontal over the eyes, or in vertex, brought on by excitement; often occurs at regular time periods of 7 or 14 days' cycle.

Digestive System. *B. Dysenteric* has been shown to have selective action on the pylorus causing spasm and retention of digested contents; dilatation of stomach; wakened at 12 midnight to I a. m. with acute pain in stomach, relieved by vomiting of a large quantity of mucous material.

In some children, diagnosed as- suffering from *congenital pyloric stenosis* considerable success has followed the use of *Dys. Co.* (Bach), which would suggest that in these cases the condition had been due to pyloric spasm rather than to congenital malformation, of the pylorus.

Duodenal ulcer often calls for the use of the nosode *Dys. Co.* (Bach) but there must always be present also evidence of nervous tension, which always precedes the physical symptom and which the patient feels and refers to his "stomach and heart area". This is in contrast to the type of duodenal ulcer found associated with the *B. Proteus,* where the nerve tension is insidious in action, unperceived by the patient, and the physical condition-the ulcer-tends to come on as a "crisis" without previous warning.

Cardio-vascular. Functional disturbance of heart action, associated with nerve tension; palpitation before important events; anticipatory discomfort in the cardiac area.

These are the outstanding symptoms found in the clinical proving of the nosode *Dys. Co.* (Bach), and you will find in them something of each of the associated remedies, *Arsen. Alb.; Argent. Nit.; Kalmia.*

SYCOTIC CO. (Paterson)

This organism is not of bacillary form but is a non-lactose fermenting coccus found in the intestinal tract. The details of this organism and the manner in which it was identified) is to be found in the original work published in the British Homsopathic Journal of April, 1933.

The keynote for the nosode *Sycotic Co.* (Paterson) is "irritability" and this has special reference to mucous and synovial membrane.

Mentals. Nervous irritability; tempery (cf. *Lycopodium);* fear of dark; of being left alone; twitching of facial muscles, blinking of eyelids.

Head. Irritation of meninges, sub-acute or chronic; headache from infection of sinuses; persistent headache-particularly in a child-which may be the prodromal sign of a tubercular meningitis (cf. *Hellebore).* Sweating of head at night, profuse.

Digestive System. Chronic irritation of the whole alimentary tract; catarrhal conditions; acute or chronic gastroenteritis in the child; loose offensive stool, excoriating (cf. *Medorrhinum);* urgent call to stool as soon as rising out of bed; constipation unusual; diarrhœa common; nausea or sickness after eating eggs (Cf. *Ferrum met.).*

Respiratory. Acute, sub-acute, chronic bronchial catarrh; catarrh of mucous membranes of nose, throat (enlarged tonsils and adenoids in child). Irritable cough at night, 2 a. m.

I regard *Sycotic co.* (Paterson) as a pre-tubercular remedy.

Circulation. Ancmia and hydrcmia, usually in the adult.

(The *Sycotic* patient is always anæmic looking, never carries much colour in the face.)

Neuro-muscular System. General rheumatic fibrositis, aggravated from dampness, alter a period of rest (Cf. *Rhus tox.).* Feet painful when walking, as if walking on loose cobble stones, pain in the me tarsal bones, fidgety feet at night in bed.

Skin. Sallow complexion, oily skill) vesicular or varicellar type of eruption on face or body : (After administration of *Sycotic Co.* (Paterson) to children, a rash varicellar in type, resembling, and often mistaken for *chicken-pox* may appear.) Warts on mucocutaneous surfaces.

Genito-urinary System. *Sycotic Co.* (Paterson) has marked action of the whole of the genito-urinary tract causing irritation of mucous membranes from the kidney to the urethral tract; albuminuria; pyelitis; cystitis; urethritis; vulvo-vaginitis; balanitis.

Female. Pain in left ovary at menstrual period; tic ovaries; tubal infection (tubercular or gonococcal); profuse leucorrhsa.

It will be evident that this coccal organism of the intestinal tract is related morphologically and clinically to the Gonococcus. Hahnemann related what he called "The Sycotic Miasm" to the disease, Gonorrhœa, but this disease is only one form of catarrhal infection of the mucous membrane of the urinary tract. There are many other non-gonorrhœal organisms associated with the symptom picture of "catarrh" and I suggest that the miasm "Sycosis" may be considered synonymous with "Catarrh". Gonorrhœa is an infection of mucous membrane (i. e. it is a sycotic manifestation) but catarrhal manifestations *(Sycotic)* are not all due to gonorrhœal infection.

These are the nosodes prepared from the non-lactose fermenting organisms of the bowel which are most generally called for in practice, but there are two other members which are found occasionally in the stool and which are not well proved and seldom used.

MUTABILE (Bach)

This bacillus is so named because it *mutates* almost as soon as it is sub-cultured from a non-lactose to a lactose fermenter and is of interest mainly from a bacteriological point of view as the *Bacillus Mutabile* is an intermediary form between the *B. Coli* and the true non-lactose fermenting type. Its associated remedy is *Pulsatilla* and the nosode *Mutabile* (Bach) is likely to be of value in treatment where there is alteration of symptoms, e. g. where skin eruption alternates with asthmatic symptoms.

FAECALIS (Bach)

I have never found this nosode made from the *B. Faecalis* of much value in treatment, but where I have found the organism in the stool, the clinical symptoms have led me to choose *Sepia* as the indicated remedy.

Biochemistry of the Bowel Organisms and their associated Remedies

I would ask you now to refer to the list before you and to note the group remedies which have been found associated with each type of non lactose fermenting organism of the bowel.

B. MORGAN (Bach)

In this group two elements are outstanding, i. e., *Sulphur* and *Carbon.* In this group also there are complex remedies from the plant world, e. g. *Lycopodium* and from the venom of a snake, i. e. *Lachesis.*

B. Proteus (Bach)

Here the outstanding element is *Chlorine.*

BACILLUS No. "7" (Paterson)

Bromine and *iodine.*

B. GAERTNER (Bach)

Silicea; Phosphorus; Fluorine; Merc. Viv.

From this list it will be evident that each organism is associated with remedies which have a central element with which other elements may combine to form remedies of varying chemical complexity. The practice of Homeopathy is founded on the hypothesis That the true *simillimum* (the homœopathic remedy) is related to the disturbed metabolism (the disease) and now it can be demonstrated that the non -lactose fermenting organism of the bowel is biochemically related to the disease and the homœopathic remedy.

The potentized vaccine -the nosode- prepared from culture of the organism can be considered to be a complex biochemical substance having the characteristic of the disturbed metabolism, and thus to be similar to the disease and according to the law of similars, to have specific therapeutic power to restore balance, a condition of ease -i. e. health.

The individual members of each group may have some therapeutic action in a specific disease, but the action of the simpler elements may be incomplete and require the assistance of the more, Complex remedies, and on this hypothesis one can formulate a series of working rules for the use of the remedies and the nosodes and in actual practice demonstrate how one may complement the action of the other.

INDICATIONS FOR THE USE OF THE BOWEL NOSODES IN DISEASE

My remarks will be addressed, on this occasion, to those doctors ho have no means of obtaining bacteriological reports on stool culture, but who may wish to try out the use of these nosodes in their practice.

I suggest that we divide the cases to be considered into two groups :

(1) ***New Case***. A patient who has *not received homś opathic treatment.*

(2) ***Old Case***. A patient who has been under homsopathic treatment but who may not be responding to the treatment given.

In using the bowel nosodes it must always be remembered that they are deep acting remedies and cover the totality of symptoms from the highest level, the "mentals", to the lowest level of gross pathology" *and* that they also cover the life history of a patient from earliest childhood to adult life or old age.

The "taking of the case history" is therefore of great importance in the choice of the nosode for a particular case, and attention must be given to the "past" as well as the "present" symptom

New Case. Where this is a definite symptom picture which points to a remedy, this should be given, and not a nosode. In many cases, how-ever, the choice may lie within a number of possible remedies and it is in this difficulty that one may use the list of remedies and the associated bowel nosodes. If; for example, *Sulphur, Calcarea Carbonica, Graphites* were among the list of possible remedies, reference to the table would show that the nosode *Morgan-pure* (Paterson) was related to each of these arid could be considered to cover the totality of the symptoms. In practice this is found to be so and proves the bowel nosodes to be deep and broad acting remedies.

As another example, the choice might lie within the group of remedies *Merc. viv., Phosphorus, Silicea,* in which case the nosode *Gaertner* (Bach) would be indicated.

In this way it is possible to choose the nosode from the list of possible remedies for a given case, but the next question to decide is that of potency and repetition of dose.

As in general homœopathic practice the more obvious the "mentals" the higher the potency, but if there are marked pathological symptoms the general rule is to employ the lower potencies.

With outstanding "mentals" I prefer the nosode in 1m potency or higher, if obtainable, but if there is obvious evidence of advanced pathological conditions such as advanced rheumatoid arthritis, or malignancy, I would employ the *6c* potency and give this in a daily dose over a period, the duration of which would be determined by clinical observation and evidence of reaction.

Between these extremes there is an intermediate level of potency -The 30C- which I have found useful where there is a combination of acute and chronic, e. g. in acute broncho-pneumonia superimposed upon a chronic condition, with a miasmatic background, a tubercular diathesis.

The number and frequency of the doses of the chosen nosode can be determined only by clinical observation and experience.

The higher the potency chosen the less frequent the repetition and number of doses, is a good working rule for the use of the nosodes, but it has been found a useful practice to complement the action of a nosode in single high potency dose, with repeated doses of the low potency of an associated remedy. As example, a case of skin eruption may call for a single dose of *Morgan-pure* (Paterson) 1M but the intolerable itch may also call for *Sulphur* in the *3X* to the 6c potency in repeated doss. Also in chronic arthritis, alter a dose of the appropriate nosode for the case, considerable benefit to the patient may follow the use of a low potency remedy, chosen from the list of associated remedies, and given over a considerable period of time.

Old Case. This is where the patient may have had homœopathic treatment over a period and received a considerable number of remedies with a varying degree of success or failure. These are difficult cases, even from the nosode point of view; when there is no evidence available from stool culture to give a clue to the group of remedies likely to be useful, or as to the phase in which the patient is at the moment. It must he remembered that the potentized remedy can alter the bowel flora and that in an "old case" the remedies already given may have caused a positive phase, i. e. changed the *B. Coli* to non-lactose fermenting bacilli, and consideration must be given to the extent of this change. If I find a percentage of non-lactose fermenting organisms in a stool greater than 50 per cent., I at once determine that the administration of a bowel nosode is contraindicated, and experience has shown that a nosode given at such a time produces a negative phase with a corresponding period of vital depression in the patient.

With this uncertainty in an old case, which has had potentized remedies within one month, it is wiser to use a nosode in the & potency in the first instance, and so avoid the chance of a violent negative reaction.

The choice of a nosode for any case can be determined by a study of the clinical history and noting the remedies which have given the greatest, although not sustained, effect. Tabulate this list of remedies and compare it with the Nosode list and the associated remedies and choose the nosode which has the greatest number within its group. In many cases there may not be much apparent effect from the nosode, but it would seem that the giving of the nosode had in some manner readjusted the case, because thereafter considerable benefit follows the remedy previously given without much effect. If there seems no apparent benefit from the nosode, do not be disappointed but repeat the remedy which has given the evidence of partial reaction before, and this time you can expect more permanent action.

One last remark, and that of warning, do not repeat a bowel nosode within three months ; but if it is necessary to prescribe, select a remedy within the group, and give the remedy in high or low potency as you find indicated from the symptoms present. Finally, do not expect too much from these bowel nosodes, and then be disappointed in their use. They are valuable therapeutic agents when properly used, and their great value is in the treatment of chronic disease, in cases which are generally considered to be very resistant to any form of treatment.

Note on Nomenclature.

3x = 3rd decimal Hahnemannian

6c = 6 centesimal Hahnemannian

30c = 30 centesimal Hahnemannian

1m = 1,000 centesimal Hahnemannian

AMENDED LIST (SEPTEMBER, 1949).

(A) *Morgan-Pure* (Paterson)	Alumina Baryta carb. Calc. carb. Calc. sulph. Carbo veg. Carbo sulph. Digitalis Ferrum carb. Medorrhinum	Graphites Kali.carb. Mag carb. Nat. carb. Petroleum Psorinum Sepia *SULPHUR* Tuberc. bov.
(B) *Morgan-Gaertner* (Paterson)	Chelidonium Chenopodium Hellebor. nig. Hepar. sulph. Lachesis	LYCOPODIUM Merc. sulph. Sanguinaria Taraxacum
PROTEUS (Bach)	Ac. mur. Amon. mur. Aurum mur. Apis Baryta mur. Borax Conium Cuprum met.	Calc. mur. Ferr. mur. Ignatia Kali. mur. Mag. mur. *NATRUM MUR.* Secale
MUTABILE (Bach)	Ferrum phos. Kali phos. Kali. sulph. *PULSATILLA*	
BACILLUS No. "7" (Paterson)	Arsen. iod. *Bromium* Calc iod. Ferrum iod. *IODUM* Kali. bich.	Kali. brom. *KALI. CARB.* Kali. nit. Merc. iod. Nat. iod.

GAERTNER (Bach)	Calc. fluor. Calc. hypophos. Calc. phos. Calc. sil. Kali. phos. *MERC. VIV.* Nat. phos.	Nat. Sil. Fluor. PHOSPHORUS Phytolacca Pulsatilla SILICEA Syphilinum Zinc. phos.
Dys. Co. (Bach)	Anacardium Argentum nit. *ARSENICUM ALB.* Cadmium met.	Kalmia Veratrum album Veratrum viride
SYCOTIC Co. (Paterson)	Ac. nit. Antim. tart. Bacillinum Calc. metal. Ferrum met.	Natrum sulph. Rhus. tox. *Thuja*
FAECALIS (Bach)	*SEPIA*	